THE INTIMATE QUESTION BOOK

222 INDISCREET AND EROTIC QUESTIONS FOR COUPLES

THE INTIMATE QUESTION BOOK

Welcome to your intimate Q&A session.

In this book, in 6 chapters, a total of 222 indiscreet questions about sexuality, love and relationships await you. It's pretty hot, because the questions are both daring and exciting. Make yourself comfortable, create a romantic or tingling atmosphere and get going.

You can ask each other the questions alternately, or both of you can answer every single question. If you prefer not to answer one or the other question, you can also choose any number of jokers before the game starts, which will allow you to keep quiet on the topic. This can even provide additional thrills. Just the way you want it. The main thing is that you have fun getting to know each other in a playful, crackling way and that you can spark the desire to play. How the question round ends is up to you.

May the erotic game begin.

Have fun!

CONTENTS

FANTASIES

What movie is playing in my mental cinema?

Do you have a fetish that you have never told anyone about before, but which you would like to live out one day?

____

____

____

____

____

____

Do certain clothes turn you on during sex? Lace, patent leather, latex?

____

____

____

____

____

What do you think about BDSM? Would you rather be dominant or submissive and where would your limits be?

____

____

____

____

____

____

Do you like porn? If so, do you have a category that particularly turns you on?

____

____

____

____

____

In which places would you like to have exciting sex?

____

____

____

____

____

____

If you could spend one night with a celebrity, who would it be?

____

____

____

____

____

Would you like to have a threesome sometime? With two women or two men?

____

____

____

____

____

____

Do you find the thought appealing that someone might be watching us have sex?

____

____

____

____

____

____

Does the thought of being caught having sex turn you on more, or is it not for you at all?

____

____

____

____

____

____

How do you feel about watching your partner having sex with others?

____

____

____

____

____

____

Do you ever think about something or someone in particular
during sex?

____

____

____

____

____

____

Does it turn you on when I masturbate in front of you or
when we masturbate together?

____

____

____

____

____

Would you like to visit a swingers club and do a partner exchange?

____

____

____

____

____

____

Do you find role playing exciting? Which scenarios and costumes particularly turn you on?

____

____

____

____

____

Food for pleasure: Exciting or a no-go?

____

____

____

____

____

____

If you could shop to your heart's content in a sex shop, what would you buy?

____

____

____

____

____

____

Would you like to be in a porn movie yourself? What genre
could you imagine?

____

____

____

____

____

____

Do you find erotic novels exciting and would you like to
write one yourself? What would it be about?

____

____

____

____

____

How would you like to go out on a frivolous date? What would you do and wear?

____

____

____

____

____

Do you find uniforms sexy? Are there any that turn you on? Why is that?

____

____

____

____

____

Angel and little devil: What do you like more? Innocent and good or evil and wild?

____

____

____

____

____

____

Is there a feature you find particularly sharp? For example, a smoky voice, a beard, a certain eye color, long hair, big breasts, a dress style?

____

____

____

____

____

____

Do you ever imagine having sex with someone you don't know? Which scenario is attractive to you? In a club, at a festival, in a bar, on a train?

____

____

____

____

____

____

Would you like to try Tantra? What do you think, does it have an effect on your and our sexuality?

____

____

____

____

____

Is blindfolded sex a fantasy that sounds tempting to you?

____

____

____

____

____

____

Where would you most like to do an erotic photo shoot? What kind of clothes and/or makeup would you wear?

____

____

____

____

____

Which toy would you like to include in sex?

____

____

____

____

____

____

You think the idea of getting a striptease is hot?

____

____

____

____

____

Do you find the idea of sleeping with a much older person interesting or rather repulsive?

____

____

____

____

____

____

Have you ever had wild sex dreams? With whom and where have you done it?

____

____

____

____

____

Have you ever thought about offering someone sex in return? Does the thought turn you on?

____

____

____

____

____

Would you like to be a nude model? Would you rather be a model for a draftsman or an erotic model for catalogues or calendars?

____

____

____

____

____

How does sex with a masked person at a masked ball sound
to you?

____

____

____

____

____

____

Do you have erotic daydreams? What do you think about?

____

____

____

____

____

____

Which position or game would you like to try out?

____

____

____

____

____

Could you imagine taking a nudist vacation?

____

____

____

____

____

Do you think it's hot to send dirty messages and pictures to each other while you're working? Or is it just distracting and should wait until after work?

Can you think of anything else about fantasies?

BODY

The physics of love

Do you have an erogenous zone I haven't heard about?

____

____

____

____

____

____

Women: Is clitoral or vaginal orgasm better for you?
Men: Do you prefer to come inside or outside the vagina?

____

____

____

____

____

____

Do you find piercings and tattoos of the genital area sexy?
Are there places, where you like them especially, or motives
you like especially? What is not possible at all?

____

____

____

____

____

Do you like the 69 position during oral sex? Do you prefer
to be up or down?

____

____

____

____

____

What do you find particularly attractive about my body?
And what about your own?

____

____

____

____

____

____

Does swallowing during oral sex turn you on?

____

____

____

____

____

____

Do you prefer to close your eyes during sex, or did you
prefer to open them?

____

____

____

____

____

Does it turn you on when things get a little wilder and, for
example, bitten, scratched and slightly pulled by your hair?

____

____

____

____

____

Do you prefer the feeling of cold or warmth during sex?
More like ice cubes, or more like wax?

____

____

____

____

____

____

Do you like anal sex and anal pampering?

____

____

____

____

____

____

Where do you first look at an attractive person?

____

____

____

____

____

How would it be for you if I/the man had starting difficulties?
How would you deal with the situation?

____

____

____

____

____

What do you consider to be part of a good foreplay? And
how long should it last?

____

____

____

____

____

____

If I let you do my makeover, how would I look afterwards?

____

____

____

____

____

____

If you could change something on your body, what would it be?

____

____

____

____

____

____

Would you ever get plastic surgery?

____

____

____

____

____

____

Do you find artificial nails, eyelashes and co. beautiful, or do you not like that about yourself/your partner at all?

____

____

____

____

____

____

What do you like more: Rather well-trained, or rather a bit chubby?

____

____

____

____

____

____

Does the size of the penis/breasts matter to you?

____

____

____

____

____

____

What does an orgasm feel like for you? Where and how do you feel it?

____

____

____

____

____

How often can you come in short intervals until you finally get enough?

____

____

____

____

____

____

What is your opinion on female ejaculation (also called squirting)? Sexy or weird?

____

____

____

____

____

Do you find sex during your period good, or would you prefer to avoid it during this time?

____

____

____

____

____

____

Would you rather have a completely different body? If so, why is that?

____

____

____

____

____

____

When did you have your first period/ejaculation?

____

____

____

____

____

____

Are you as much into giving oral sex as you are getting it?
What do you particularly like about spoiling me with your
mouth?

____

____

____

____

____

____

If I want to seduce you, what do I have to do to get you going? Are there certain parts of your body or actions that particularly spark your lust?

____

____

____

____

____

Would you like to try body painting? Would you rather be the person who paints, or the person who is painted? Which motif would you choose?

____

____

____

____

____

Do you think men and women should shave? If so, both or just the woman? Where can there be hair for you and where do you not like it at all?

____

____

____

____

____

____

Makeup, perfume, aftershave, solarium: Do you prefer me natural or do you like me with some support from the beauty industry? How much is too much of a good thing?

____

____

____

____

____

What part of your body would you like to make a mold of me? What would you do with it when it's done?

____

____

____

____

____

____

Is there a difference for you between "being aroused in the head" and "being physically aroused"? How is it different and how do you feel it? Is both equally important for you?

____

____

____

____

____

____

Do you find it disgusting to kiss after oral sex, or is it something beautiful for you that goes with it?

____

____

____

____

____

____

How wet do you think a kiss should be? And how much tongue is involved?

____

____

____

____

____

What would you find more erotic? Naked photos of me, or photos with sexy lingerie that leaves room for fantasy?

____

____

____

____

____

____

What difference does it make to you as a man/woman if we use a condom during sex? Does it feel very different?

____

____

____

____

____

Ejaculate onto the body of your partner: Exciting finale or no-go?

____

____

____

____

____

____

Can you think of anything else about the body?

____

____

____

____

____

RELATIONS

How do I define my partnership?

Would you ever consider an open relationship?

____

____

____

____

____

____

How do you think the sex has developed since we started dating?

____

____

____

____

____

Would you tell me if you were cheating or keep quiet? Why?
And what would you expect me to do in a situation like this?

Could you ever forgive a fling?

At what point would you say it's cheating? Is it still okay to
flirt, or is it too much?

____

____

____

____

____

____

Is there anything you would like in our relationship?

____

____

____

____

____

What was the best sex we had together for you? You think
we can top that?

____

____

____

____

____

In which situations do you get jealous and how do you
react?

____

____

____

____

____

What makes me different from a person you just find
sexually attractive?

____

____

____

____

____

____

Do you think that sex between two people becomes more
boring and uninteresting over time, or do you think lust can
be rekindled again and again?

____

____

____

____

____

____

Are you embarrassed when I talk about our sex with friends?

____

____

____

____

____

Do you talk to friends about sex? And if so, what do you talk about and what are your limits?

____

____

____

____

____

Do you think one should also have some secrets in a
relationship, or should one always be 100% open with each
other? What would be an unbearable secret for you, what
would be okay?

____

____

____

____

____

Does it scratch your ego when I use toys and masturbate
instead of sleeping with you? Or do you find it normal,
varied and maybe even sexy?

____

____

____

____

____

Do you prefer me to be submissive or controlling during sex?

____

____

____

____

____

____

Are you more into the cuddle sex, or is it when things get really rough?

____

____

____

____

____

____

Would you prefer a quickie or an extensive pampering
session with me?

____

____

____

____

____

____

Would you rather have sex after you get up, or before you
go to bed?

____

____

____

____

____

Is there something you've never dared to tell me but always wanted to say?

____

____

____

____

____

____

Would you prefer a classic date with me, or an erotic one?

____

____

____

____

____

Sex after a fight: energetic love affair or completely wrong
time?

If we can't see each other, would phone sex and
masturbating together be something for you?

What is for you the difference between lust and love? Can you separate them?

____

____

____

____

____

____

Do you prefer to seduce me, or would you rather be seduced by me?

____

____

____

____

____

____

Do you think age matters, or is it just a matter of love?

____

____

____

____

____

____

Do you think you have to love yourself to be able to love
really deeply? Do you love yourself?

____

____

____

____

____

____

Why did you decide for a relationship and not for a life as a single with all freedoms?

____

____

____

____

____

____

How important is fidelity in a relationship to you? Is it the be-all and end-all, or are there more important things? For example, what would that be?

____

____

____

____

____

____

Have you ever been cheated on? How did you find out
about it and what impact has it had on you and your life?

____

____

____

____

____

____

What do you need to be able to let yourself go completely
during sex?

____

____

____

____

____

What do you think: Why do people become unfaithful? Does infidelity always mean directly that the relationship is no longer working?

Do you believe in love at first sight and eternal love? Can couples be in love all their lives?

Is tenderness or sexuality more important to you in a
relationship?

____

____

____

____

____

____

How would you handle it if one of us had a sexual
preference that the other did not share? Would you try to
find a solution or a compromise, or would you ignore it and
check it off?

____

____

____

____

____

Do you think white lies are okay in a relationship? What is a white lie for you and when does it start to cross that line?

____

____

____

____

____

____

What would you do if I had a fight with your best friend? Would you stay out of it, stay neutral and express your own opinion, or would you side with one of us? Who would that be rather and why?

____

____

____

____

____

Do you ever have fear of loss? When do these occur and
how do you deal with them? Are there any situations that
are particularly sensitive for you?

____

____

____

____

____

Can you think of anything else about relationships?

____

____

____

____

____

EXPERIENCES

What have I experienced and
what has shaped me?

Have you ever had a one-night stand? What did you think?

____

____

____

____

____

____

Have you ever had a friendship plus? How did that change
the friendship?

____

____

____

____

____

____

How many people have you had sex with?

____

____

____

____

____

Have you ever had something with a person and regretted it afterwards? Why did you regret it?

____

____

____

____

____

Have you ever done something with someone that you haven't tried with me? Would you like to do it again?

____

____

____

____

____

____

Have you ever paid someone an allowance for sex or had yourself paid an allowance? How did it come about and what was it like?

____

____

____

____

____

How was your first time? Was it better or worse than expected?

How old were you when you first came?

What was the most embarrassing thing that ever happened
to you during sex and what happened afterwards?

Have you ever been involved with a person you should have
stayed away from? A teacher, best friend's girlfriend, a
doctor?

Have you ever had a multiple orgasm? How did it feel for
you?

____

____

____

____

____

____

Have you ever been caught having sex? By whom and
where?

____

____

____

____

____

Has anyone ever crossed your intimate threshold? What happened and how did you react?

____

____

____

____

____

____

Have you ever faked an orgasm? What made you do that?

____

____

____

____

____

Have you ever said you were taken even though you were single, just to get away from a person who was not your type?

____

____

____

____

____

____

Have you ever been given a wrong phone number? Did it make you laugh, or did it offend you?

____

____

____

____

____

Have you ever used your male/female advantages to get out
of a situation better or to gain advantages? What was the
situation and what did you do?

____

____

____

____

____

What is the most extraordinary, funniest or most exciting
place you have ever had sex? Was this a spontaneous idea
or planned?

____

____

____

____

____

What have you done that you used to think you would never do? In retrospect, were you happy to have done it after all, or would you have preferred to stick to your principle?

____

____

____

____

____

Have you ever had to stop sex because you needed to go to the bathroom? Were you embarrassed?

____

____

____

____

____

Have you ever had a disaster date that went completely different than expected? What happened?

When you were in school, did you ever secretly give someone a gift for Valentine's Day without that person knowing who it came from?

Have you ever called a sex hotline for real or fun?

____

____

____

____

____

____

What was your craziest chat experience? What was your most embarrassing?

____

____

____

____

____

Have you ever sent naked pictures of yourself to anyone?
Have you ever regretted it?

Have you ever been in love with a teacher? How old were
you and how did you deal with the situation?

Who was your first crush generally? How old were you then?

____

____

____

____

____

____

Have you ever been in a totally inappropriate situation?
What kind of situation was that and how did you deal with
it?

____

____

____

____

____

Have you ever sent a salacious message to the wrong person? What happened and who was the person?

What was the meanest or most unexpected rejection you ever received? Did it make you doubt yourself, or did you deal with it casually, since you can't and don't have to please everyone?

Have you ever deflowered anyone?

____

____

____

____

____

____

Have you ever had sex dreams with a person you would never do anything with in real life?

____

____

____

____

____

What crazy and permissive party games have you played
and how far have you gone?

____

____

____

____

____

____

Have you ever had sex so loud that the neighbours
complained?

____

____

____

____

____

Have you ever had to see a doctor about a sex accident?
What happened?

____

____

____

____

____

____

Have you ever watched someone having sex secretly? How
did it happen and were you discovered?

____

____

____

____

____

Have you ever had sex while other people were in the
room? Did they notice any of this?

Can you think of anything else about experiences?

SEXUAL IDENTITY

Who am I and how do I perceive
myself as man or woman?

Have you ever had fantasies or experiences with the same sex? What was it like for you?

____

____

____

____

____

When do you think you'll really be old enough for sex?

____

____

____

____

____

Do you think it's good that gays and lesbians can get married and adopt children? Why do you have that opinion?

____

____

____

____

____

____

Was there a time in your life when you wished you were the opposite sex? How did it come about and how long did this phase last?

____

____

____

____

____

____

What makes you feel male/female? Is there something for you that is typically male/female?

____

____

____

____

____

____

Are you comfortable in your role as man/woman?

____

____

____

____

____

____

How often do you need and want to have sex so that you can feel fullfilled?

How often do you satisfy yourself? Has it become less since we've been together, or have you maintained that frequency?

Do you find it brave or embarrassing when people dress and wear make-up like the opposite sex?

____

____

____

____

____

____

Do you have male/female parts in you? When do they come out?

____

____

____

____

____

Do you think that men and women should be treated equally on every point, or are there exceptions?

____

____

____

____

____

____

Do you think we humans are monogamous by nature or is fidelity just a socially imposed rule?

____

____

____

____

____

____

Should the man make the first step, or is it a matter of both sexes?

____

____

____

____

____

____

When did you realize that you would like to have your first time and that you are ready for it? How did that happen?

____

____

____

____

____

How did you get enlightened? Did you make an effort to expand your knowledge in the field yourself, for example by reading magazines or exchanging information with older friends?

____

____

____

____

____

Do you think gender reassignment is a good thing for transgender people, or do you think everyone should live as he/she was born and accept it?

____

____

____

____

____

Sigmund Freud was of the opinion that every person is secretly bisexually inclined. You think there's something to that, or is that bullshit?

More and more terms for sexual orientation and gender are appearing in the media. Do you think there is more than heterosexual and homosexual and male and female? Or are these just trend words for you?

How would you support and help a friend when he/she
wants to come out but is afraid of the reactions of others?

____

____

____

____

____

____

Do you think that sexual interests and orientations can
change in the course of a person's life? In what respect?

____

____

____

____

____

Do you think homosexual couples have less misunderstandings and better sex because they are of the same sex and know what the other one needs? Or is that a cliché?

How would you feel about not having sex until after the wedding? Do you think that can have positive sides or are you even a supporter?

Do you ever wonder what sex feels like for the opposite sex?
Do you think men or women have more fun and more
intense orgasms? Or is it equally nice for both?

Would you like to go to a cross-dressing party where people
consciously dress like the opposite sex? What would you be
attracted to and what would you wear?

What do you think are the three biggest advantages of
being a man, what are the three biggest advantages of
being a woman?

____

____

____

____

____

____

When should children be educated at school? Should this be
done by the teachers, or a professional team from an
organisation or similar?

____

____

____

____

____

Should children and young people be taught that sexual orientations other than heterosexual and other genders than male and female are also normal, or do you think this goes too far?

____

____

____

____

____

Do you think women have it harder in the working world? In what way and why is that? How could the problem be solved or at least the situation improved?

____

____

____

____

____

Men bring the money home, women take care of the household. Do you think there's any truth to this cliché, or is it a long outdated role model?

What should men and women finally know and understand in relation to the opposite sex? What are points that in your opinion always lead to misunderstandings? Do we have such points?

Is there anything that should remain purely male or female domain for you? What is that and why do you feel that way?

____

____

____

____

____

____

Do you think contraception is just a women's issue, or is it an issue that concerns both?

____

____

____

____

____

Is there anything that makes you doubt yourself as a man/woman? What helps you at a time like this?

____

____

____

____

____

____

What do you think about the fact that in society and advertising, for example, girls are identified with the colour pink, ballet and horses and boys with the colour blue, football and dinosaurs? Should children be free to choose?

____

____

____

____

____

Do you think that girls-only or boys-only schools will lead to problems of identity and sexuality for the children later on? Do you believe that these children and teenagers will later lack something?

____

____

____

____

____

Do you prefer friends of the same sex or the opposite sex? Is there a particular reason for this?

____

____

____

____

____

Are women during their periods and men during a cold really that bad? Do you think that's true for us too? Which one of us gets more worked up in a situation like this?

____

____

____

____

____

Can you think of anything else about sexual identity?

____

____

____

____

____

MORALS AND LIMITS

Where does the fun end?

Where do you stand on prostitution? Good cause, or should it be illegal?

____

____

____

____

____

____

Do you think that pornography has a negative effect on the image of women and men, sexuality and even relationships?

____

____

____

____

____

Consensual sex with violence and pain: sick fetish, which you strictly reject, or forbidden fruit, which sounds tempting?

____

____

____

____

____

____

Have you ever used it to your advantage that a person was very drunk? What did you do?

____

____

____

____

____

Do you find it reprehensible or acceptable when people are together and marry only for financial reasons?

____

____

____

____

____

____

What do you think: Is the person who starts something with a forgiven or married person just as guilty, or is the responsibility entirely on the unfaithful partner?

____

____

____

____

____

____

Do you think a person who once cheated will always cheat? Or can it vary from relationship to relationship?

____

____

____

____

____

____

If you fall in love with another person while in a relationship, should you tell your partner or keep it a secret to protect the relationship?

____

____

____

____

____

If you found out that your best friend was cheating, would you cover for him/her in front of your partner, or would you get involved and persuade him/her to tell the truth before you did?

____

____

____

____

____

Men who have had many sexual partners are Casanovas. Women who have had many sexual partners are sluts. Do you agree with the common cliché or do you disagree?

____

____

____

____

____

Do you think it's okay to flirt and hire strippers at the bachelor party again, or should you hold back on that day too, since you're in a committed relationship?

____

____

____

____

____

Does it make the situation worse or better if a fling happened while drunk? Can alcohol make you do something you will regret afterwards, or is that not a reason for such a slip?

____

____

____

____

____

What is an absolute taboo subject for you? What would you never want to try or be able to tolerate in other people? What would you do if you saw such a situation?

____

____

____

____

____

Have you ever violated your own principles? How did it come about and what was the situation? Did you regret it afterwards, or was it worth it?

____

____

____

____

____

What do you think would be an appropriate punishment for sex offenders? Are such people too much protected by the law so far?

____

____

____

____

____

____

Is the ex-girlfriend of a boyfriend or girlfriend taboo, or is it okay to do something with him or her?

____

____

____

____

____

Is it possible to demand an HIV test and a test for sexually transmitted diseases from your partner before you have sex for the first time together, or do you think this is transnational?

____

____

____

____

____

How do you like it when couples go to the bathroom in front of each other? Is that a sign of trust, or should at least that remain intimate in a relationship and take place behind closed doors?

____

____

____

____

____

Is it okay for you to talk to your friends about when and what we are arguing about? Or do you think it's just between you and me?

____

____

____

____

____

____

How do you feel about sleeping your way up the corporate ladder? Reprehensible or useful when you might even find the person attractive and single?

____

____

____

____

____

What do you think of women who let themselves be bought drinks even though they have no interest in men? And how do you feel about men who pretend to understand women just to get a woman into bed?

____

____

____

____

____

A woman who has dressed very sexy is sexually harassed: Is it only the perpetrator's fault, or is the woman partly to blame, because she provoked with her outfit? What about an outdoor pool, sauna or nudist beach?

____

____

____

____

____

You see in public a couple where the girl is clearly underage and the man is much older. How do you react? Do you interfere?

____

____

____

____

____

____

Should it always be the man who pays for a date, or is that an old-fashioned view?

____

____

____

____

____

Persuading your partner to have sex even though he or she does not really feel like it: Are you okay with that, or should a no be accepted?

____

____

____

____

____

____

Is sex in public a tingly experience, or something you find reprehensible?

____

____

____

____

____

Should pedophiles be allowed to be castrated? What about those who were wrongly convicted?

____

____

____

____

____

____

When you realize that you don't love someone anymore, should you be honest directly, or wait and see if the feelings change again and this is just a phase?

____

____

____

____

____

____

Is it okay to go on vacation as a woman with your best friend or as a man with your best friend?

____

____

____

____

____

____

Do you find it flattering that I'm jealous, or does it annoy you more? What's the limit to where it tips over?

____

____

____

____

____

____

Is breaking up via SMS, WhatsApp or phone okay and maybe even normal in this day and age, or is it not possible at all?

____

____

____

____

____

____

Is it reprehensible to expose an ex-partner as unfaithful at the request of the new partner when he or she asks about the reason for separation?

____

____

____

____

____

Is it okay to watch porn while in a relationship?

____

____

____

____

____

____

How do you feel about keeping things from your ex-partner
despite new relationship?

____

____

____

____

____

And what about being friends with your ex-partner even though you are in a new relationship?

____

____

____

____

____

____

Is it the decision of both partners whether to keep the child, or does the woman have the right to decide alone, as it is her body?

____

____

____

____

____

Can one love too much? And should both love each other
equally in a partnership so that it works?

____

____

____

____

____

____

Can you think of anything else about morality and
boundaries?

____

____

____

____

____

Publisher: © ANGRON GmbH, Würmstr. 55, 82166 Gräfelfing, Germany

Credits: © Depositphotos / KateNovikova, Marchi, glorcza